YOUR
10-MINUTE
WELLNESS
JOURNAL

First published in Great Britain in 2024 by
Michael O'Mara Books Limited
9 Lion Yard
Tremadoc Road
London SW4 7NQ

A CIP catalogue record for this book is available from the British Library.

This product is made of material from well-managed, FSC®-certified forests and other controlled sources. The manufacturing processes conform to the environmental regulations of the country of origin.

ISBN: 978-1-78929-616-7 in paperback print format

1 2 3 4 5 6 7 8 9 10

Cover design by Jade Wheaton using an illustration
by Lee Foster-Wilson licensed by Jehane Ltd.
Designed by Jade Wheaton
Illustrations © Lee Foster-Wilson Licensed by Jehane Ltd.

Printed and bound in China

This book contains advice which is for guidance only and should not be relied upon as an alternative to professional advice from either your doctor or a registered specialist. You are strongly recommended to consult a doctor if you have any medical or other physical concerns. Neither the publisher nor the author can accept any responsibility for any consequences that may follow if such specialist advice is not sought.

www.mombooks.com

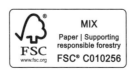

MIX
Paper | Supporting
responsible forestry
FSC® C010256

YOUR
10-MINUTE
WELLNESS
JOURNAL

Simple Exercises to Reconnect
Your Mind, Body and Soul

GILL THACKRAY

ILLUSTRATED BY LEE FOSTER-WILSON

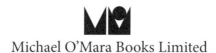

Michael O'Mara Books Limited

Introduction

Do you want to figure out how to deal with stress,
uncertainty, sleepless nights and burnout? What if you
could radiate with wellness, breaking free from survival
mode and the pressures of modern life? *Your 10-Minute
Wellness Journal* is your transformational toolkit, helping
you to consciously shift from overwhelm to calm. Explore
your own unique ecosystem of mind, body and soul
using effective tools and techniques to manifest a life
of extraordinary wellbeing.

Use this journal to awaken your wellness potential using
the prompts, reflections and guided exercises. Tune into
the interconnectedness of all living things using tried-
and-tested techniques to bring you back to oneness.
Lean into centuries-old mystical practices to achieve
life-changing spiritual and emotional balance.

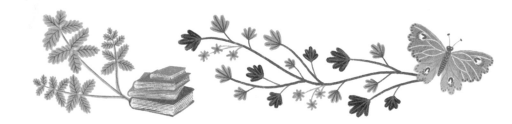

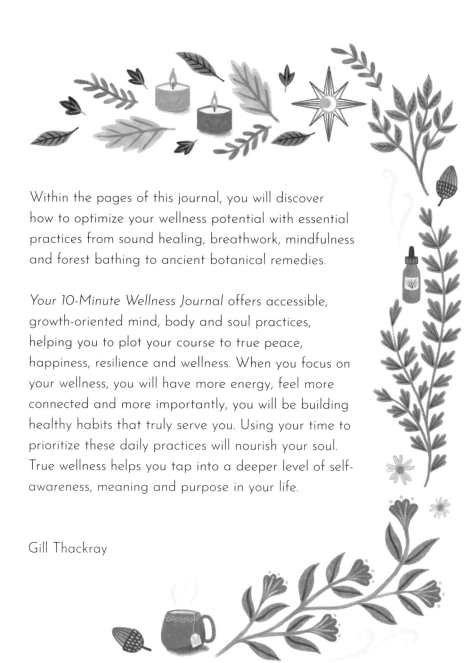

Within the pages of this journal, you will discover how to optimize your wellness potential with essential practices from sound healing, breathwork, mindfulness and forest bathing to ancient botanical remedies.

Your 10-Minute Wellness Journal offers accessible, growth-oriented mind, body and soul practices, helping you to plot your course to true peace, happiness, resilience and wellness. When you focus on your wellness, you will have more energy, feel more connected and more importantly, you will be building healthy habits that truly serve you. Using your time to prioritize these daily practices will nourish your soul. True wellness helps you tap into a deeper level of self-awareness, meaning and purpose in your life.

Gill Thackray

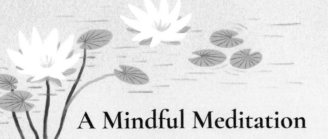

A Mindful Meditation

When you're feeling stressed, anxious or at the precipice of overwhelm, focusing on your breath is one of the quickest ways to centre yourself. There is a growing body of research to suggest that mindful meditation reduces stress, depression and anxiety. Meditation will release you from the grip of negative emotions, allowing you to step into your personal power, remaining relaxed, calm, and ready for what life brings.

1. Sit or lie down in a comfortable position. Close your eyes or leave them open, whichever feels most comfortable.

2. Begin by taking three deep breaths, in and out. On each out breath, see if it's possible to relax a little more each time.

3. Invite yourself to focus on the sensations of each breath. What do you notice as you breathe in?

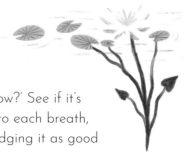

4. Ask yourself: 'What's here for me, right now?' See if it's possible to bring an attitude of curiosity to each breath, accepting whatever you notice without judging it as good or bad.

5. If your mind wanders, which it will, notice and bring your focus back to your breath. If it happens again, that's OK.

6. Continue until ten minutes has passed.

How I feel afterwards

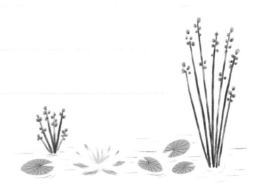

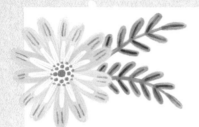

Cultivating Gratitude

There are some days when positivity feels like feels like a Sisyphean task. Uninvited challenges can leave us feeling fragile. During times like these, focusing on what we are grateful for changes our internal landscape. Researchers at Penn University found that the simple act of cultivating gratitude changes your brain, reducing toxic emotions, stress, anxiety and depression. Dr Robert Emmons from the University of California lays out three steps to gratitude. At the end of each day, use these steps to reflect on what you are grateful for.

Step 1: Recognition. I am grateful for

1. ....

2. ....

3. ....

Step 2: Acknowledgement. The good things in my life are

1. ....

2. ....

3. ....

Step 3: Appreciation. I can extend gratitude to myself for

1. ....

2. ....

3. ....

Boost Your Confidence

Developing your confidence is a wellness superpower. Researchers at the University of Dundee found a key link between self-confidence and mental health. Developing confidence is a powerful process that helps us to build more positive stories about ourselves and the world.

Setting yourself simple goals and monitoring your progress along the way is an effective tool to build self-confidence. When you start to believe in yourself, your aspirations will begin to expand. You will find yourself stepping out of the shadows, setting more ambitious goals, and interacting with the world in a more hopeful way.

Three positive things about myself

1.

2.

3.

The goals that I will set for the next month are

1.

2.

3.

I can develop positive self-talk around my goals by

1.

2.

3.

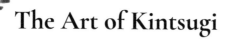

The Art of Kintsugi

The centuries-old Japanese art form of *kintsugi*, meaning 'golden joinery', repairs cracked, flawed and damaged ceramics with a lacquer mixed with powdered gold, silver or platinum. Instead of being diminished by their imperfections, these works of art are highly prized, epitomizing the philosophy of *mottainai*, a sense of regret over waste.

The concept of *kintsugi* can be extended to the challenges of life – even negative experiences are not to be wasted because they can help us to learn. Embracing and reframing bitter experiences is an effective strategy in your wellness first-aid kit. From these testing experiences, we can create something new and find strength and resilience in our vulnerability.

The challenges I have faced and overcome

_____

_____

_____

The beauty that I can create from that is

_____

_____

_____

From those experiences I learned that my strengths are

_____

_____

_____

Create Your Own Calm

Although experiencing stress is a normal part of life, sometimes it feels overwhelming. When that happens, the brain perceives danger, secreting hormones such as adrenaline and cortisol. Known as fight-or-flight, this state of arousal drains our energy, negatively impacting our health and wellbeing. Cultivating a sense of calm will help you to navigate stressful events with greater skill.

Professor Herbert Benson at Harvard Medical School demonstrated that calming strategies, such as diaphragmatic breathing, soothe the brain, supporting the body's 'rest and digest' mode, helping us to come back into a relaxed state.

Diaphragmatic breathing, which involves breathing deep into the stomach and fully engaging the diaphragm, will dial down internal stress, reduce your blood pressure, and activate your parasympathetic nervous system, restoring calm.

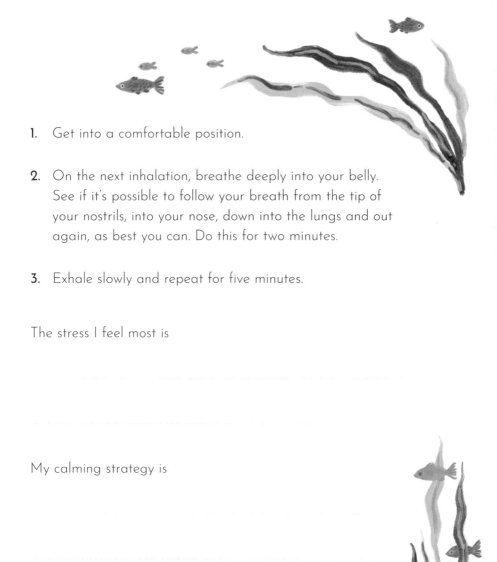

1. Get into a comfortable position.

2. On the next inhalation, breathe deeply into your belly. See if it's possible to follow your breath from the tip of your nostrils, into your nose, down into the lungs and out again, as best you can. Do this for two minutes.

3. Exhale slowly and repeat for five minutes.

The stress I feel most is

My calming strategy is

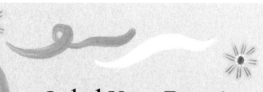

Label Your Emotions

Have you ever felt as though you were so deeply in the grip of stress that you just couldn't think clearly? That's the part of the brain called the amygdala, the processing centre for our emotions. It can cloud our ability to self-regulate. Labelling and reframing your emotions interrupts what is known as the 'stress circuit' or 'feedback loop' of stress.

When we remove the negative narrative around stress, we take away the emotional cause of fight-or-flight, stopping those toxic stress hormones, such as cortisol and adrenaline, in their tracks. That shifts the activity to the prefrontal cortex, otherwise known as the CEO of the brain. That's the part that processes information effectively, helping us to make good decisions. Labelling our emotions enables us to self-regulate the next time we are in the grip of stress.

Label your emotions. Acknowledge the feeling rather than being defined by it.

I feel

Reframe the emotion. For example, anxious thoughts could be transformed into feeling excited.

I feel

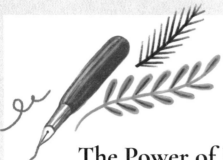

The Power of Periodization

Do you ever have days where you tackle one stressful task after another? That's the enemy of wellness and the road to burnout. This is where periodization – which is the planned division of training into separate phases – comes in. Traditionally used by athletes, the origins of this wellness-supporting performance hack are in sports psychology. Periodization will help you to dial down daily stress by identifying and managing busy tasks. You can incorporate this resilience-building strategy into your life to manage your energy levels throughout the day.

1. Where are the peaks and troughs of activity in your day? Create a list of tasks for your day.

2. Now, sort each task into high-intensity, medium-intensity, and low-intensity categories.

3. You are going to plan your day in terms of task intensity. When you complete an intense task, follow it with a less demanding one, or if your energy reserves are totally drained, take a break.

4. If you recognize that you have a natural energy dip in the day, schedule low-focus, low-intensity tasks for that period.

My daily planner

My low-intensity tasks

My medium-intensity tasks

My high-intensity tasks

My periodization planner

	High-intensity tasks	Medium-intensity tasks
Monday		
Tuesday		
Wednesday		
Thursday		
Friday		
Saturday		
Sunday		

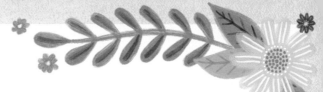

Low-intensity tasks   Order/time I will do each task

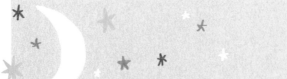

Finding Happiness

Researchers at the University of California, Berkeley have found that when we're happy we experience a whole raft of physiological benefits: our immune system becomes stronger; our blood pressure decreases; we increase our chances of improving our overall wellbeing and we reduce our stress levels. We're also more likely to make others happy simply by being around them.

You might be surprised to learn that it's not material possessions that make us happy. Consider what brings you happiness. For example, friendships and deep connections with others, hobbies, or self-care. How can you build them into your daily routine?

I am at my happiest when

I can include this in my day, week, month or year by

I can engage in random acts of kindness by

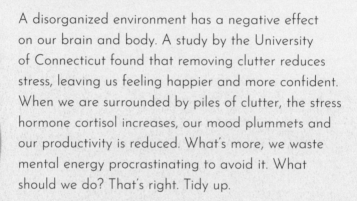

De-stress and Declutter

A disorganized environment has a negative effect on our brain and body. A study by the University of Connecticut found that removing clutter reduces stress, leaving us feeling happier and more confident. When we are surrounded by piles of clutter, the stress hormone cortisol increases, our mood plummets and our productivity is reduced. What's more, we waste mental energy procrastinating to avoid it. What should we do? That's right. Tidy up.

Start with a plan and decide which room you will begin with. For each item, the key questions are: 'Do I love it?' and 'When did I last use it?' Once you've done that, decide to donate, recycle, or organize.

Donate

What can you give to charity that you no longer use or need?
For example, clothes, jewellery, appliances, toys, or books that
you no longer want. Find a local charity with a cause close
to your heart and donate any items that might be of use to
someone else.

Items I will donate are

Recycle

Items that can be recycled are paper, electronic equipment,
glass, bulbs, plastic, or batteries. Check to see where you can
find recycling facilities in your community.

Items I will recycle

Organize

Rethink how you store your items. Is there a more efficient way to organize your clothes and other belongings? Would you benefit from storage containers, baskets or drawer dividers to store things more neatly?

Items I will keep are

I will organize these items by

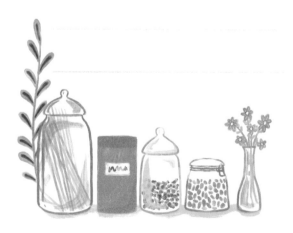

Keeping on top of your freshly organized space is
easier when you schedule a regular time to declutter.

The ways I can stay organized are

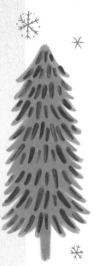

Take Time for Sisu

Finland regularly tops the United Nation's World Happiness Index. The Finnish concept of *sisu* is often credited with being the cornerstone of the nation's happiness. Rooted in the country's harsh natural environment, *sisu* means fortitude, resilience, inner strength and continued determination despite what life throws at you.

Research shows that resilience positively correlates with happiness. When we face setbacks and challenges head on, we recover from adversity quicker. You can cultivate this action-oriented Nordic trait to help you when you need to dig deep by embracing *sisu*.

I will set a daily intention to embrace *sisu* by

I will focus on what I can control by

I will continue to build my resilience by

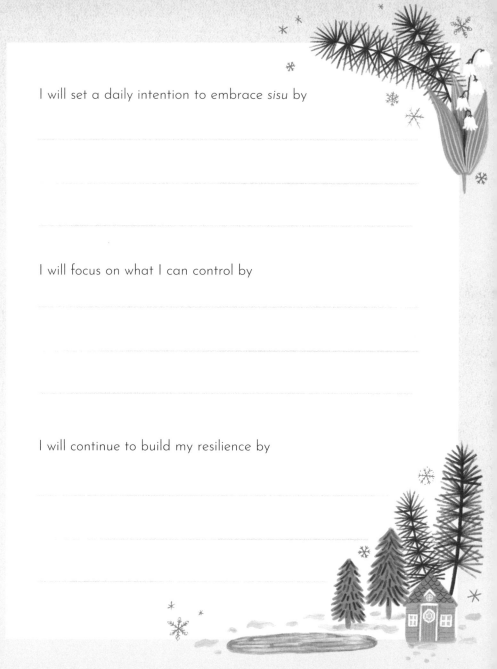

Digital Downtime

Constant digital connection can take a toll on your wellness. Mindless scrolling and persistent comparing yourself to others on social media can wear you down and impact your self-esteem, leaving you feeling 'less than'. Studies at California State University have found that digital downtime reduces stress and anxiety.

You don't need to give up all contact with the outside world. It's possible to reduce the amount of time spent online by being intentional in your use of technology. Set an 'internet-free' time to disconnect from your devices whenever you can. Begin with ten-minute blocks of tech-free time and slowly increase from there.

I will mute these email and app alerts

The apps that I no longer need are

When I do scroll, I'll do it mindfully by

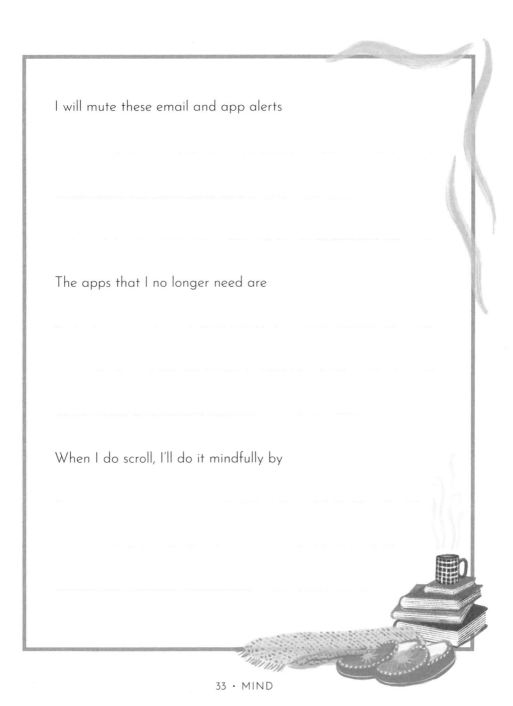

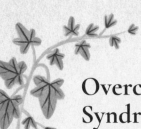

Overcoming Imposter Syndrome

Clinical psychologists Pauline Rose Clance and Suzanne Times found that imposter syndrome, the feeling that you don't deserve success and are going to be 'found out', affects one in seven of us. It's the inner critic that leaves you feeling like a fraud and full of self-doubt.

When imposter syndrome begins to stifle your growth, telling you not to step outside of your comfort zone, you can overcome it by acknowledging what you do well. The more you step outside of your comfort zone, the more your confidence and belief in yourself will flourish.

My accomplishments so far are

1.

2.

3.

I can adopt a positive mindset by

1.

2.

3.

I could accept these challenges (even if I feel the fear)

1.

2.

3.

Say 'No' with Confidence

Researchers at Safarik University, Slovenia have found that assertiveness is associated with increased self-esteem and social efficacy. Imagine this as saying 'yes' to your own needs and self-care.

When we are assertive, we can speak our truth, ask for what we want and express ourselves effectively. The ability to say 'no' clearly and calmly is a crucial wellness tool. Moreover, researchers at the University of Iowa demonstrate that we can all learn to be assertive and say 'no', however impossible it might feel. Step fully into your power by developing your assertiveness.

I can say 'no' with confidence by

_____

_____

_____

I can set boundaries with others by

_____

_____

_____

If I feel anxious about being assertive, I will calm myself by

_____

_____

_____

The Power of Positive Affirmations

Sometimes our self-talk is less than kind. These automatic, hypercritical thoughts produce a negative energy, sabotaging our potential. Affirmations are powerful tools that rewire the brain for personal and professional success, taking advantage of the brain's ability to adapt (otherwise known as neuroplasticity). Affirmations create a mindset that is supercharged for success because the conscious conversations we have with ourselves can be life changing. Create your own affirmations, targeted to areas where you recognize habitual negative thinking. State them in the present tense and repeat them daily to see your confidence soar.

- I am loved.

- I am kind and compassionate to myself and others.

- I accept myself without judgement.

- I send positive energy out into the world.

I am

I can

I accept

I embrace

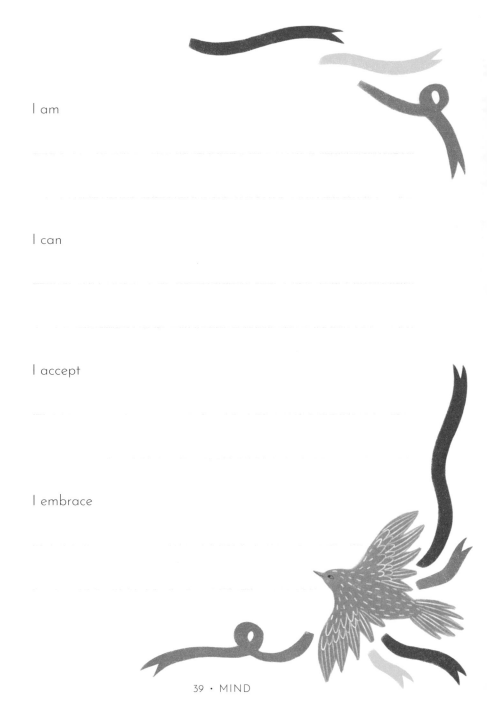

Make Time for Social Connection

Connecting with others is one of the most powerful ways of protecting ourselves against stress. Linked to improved physical and emotional wellbeing, meaningful social connections are vital for a healthy, happy life. Positive psychologist Martin Seligman found that people were happier when they had stronger social connections and less happy when those positive connections were missing. What's more, noticing and savouring the moments of positive interaction can help us to flourish. Where are the opportunities to increase your social connections?

A positive interaction I had recently was

I can reconnect with family and friends by

A group or class that I'd like to join is

I will help my community by

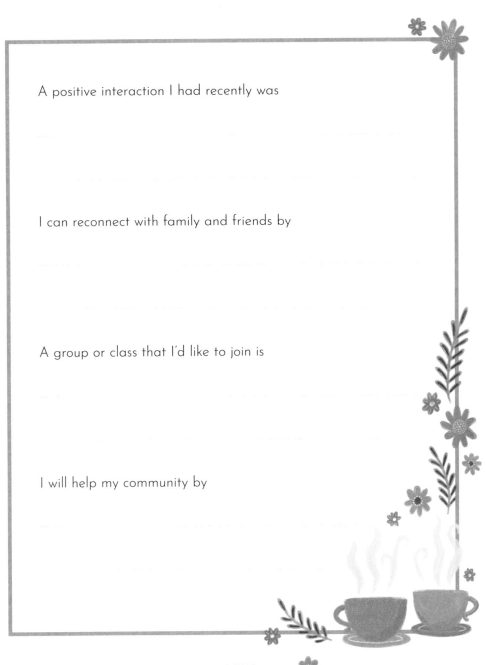

Make Change with Microhabits

Sometimes a complete health overhaul can feel overwhelming, so we don't try. The key is to start small. Forget long-term goals. Instead, break them down into microhabits. Decades of research demonstrates that breaking down your goals into smaller components and tracking your progress is enormously helpful when you want to positively change your behaviour.

These small steps will pave the way for cultivating successful change and healthy new habits. For example, taking the stairs instead of the elevator, or waking up fifteen minutes early to meditate, or setting an intention for a positive day. Take it one day at a time until you have achieved what you set out to. Celebrate your success and then create another incremental goal.

The changes I want to make in my life are

1.

2.

3.

4.

5.

These goals are important to me because

My goal hierarchy (1 being the priority and 5 being the least urgent) would be

1.

2.

3.

4.

5.

Looking at number 1, I can break this goal down into smaller, incremental goals by

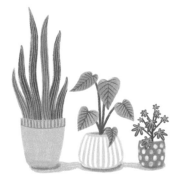

Small changes I can make to my life are

1.

2.

3.

4.

5.

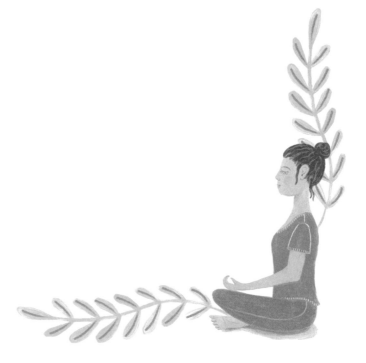

Refresh with Ayurvedic Dry Brushing

In the ancient Indian healing system of Ayurveda, balance is key. Garshana, or dry skin brushing, helps to stimulate and exfoliate the largest organ of our body, the skin. This cleansing and detoxifying practice stimulates the lymphatic system, helping to move accumulated toxins out of the body. Moreover, embarking on a dry brushing routine is a wonderful way to energize and invigorate your mind and body at the beginning of each day before a bath or shower. You will need a dry skin brush.

1. Begin with the soles of your feet, using a gentle, sweeping, upward motion.

2. Continue moving up each leg, brushing towards your heart.

3. When you arrive at your abdomen, sweep in a clockwise motion, moving upward. Notice how it feels.

4. Once you reach your arms begin with the palms of your hands, moving toward your lower arms followed by the upper arms.

5. Rinse off in the shower.

Before I begin my garshana I feel

Afterwards I feel

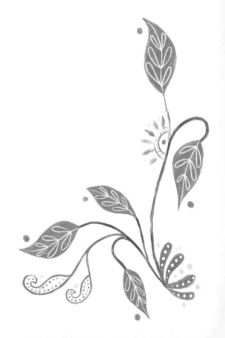

Soothe Yourself with EFT

Emotional Freedom Technique (EFT) is a powerful mind-body practice. With roots in ancient Chinese medicine, EFT is used to dispel stress by unblocking stagnant energy in the body. Thought to relieve stress, anxiety and physical pain, this simple technique involves tapping energy meridian points on the body with your fingertips.

Tapping the energy meridians (the side of the hand, sometimes called the karate chop, the crown of your head, the eyebrows, the sides of the eyes, under the eyes, under the nose, the chin, collarbone and under the arms) is believed to activate the parasympathetic nervous system, the part of the brain that controls our ability to relax and move out of fight or flight mode, dampening activity in the amygdala and reinstating calm. Here's how.

1. When you feel stressed or anxious, focus on your breath and ground yourself by staying connected to the present moment. Ask yourself, 'What do I need right now?'

2. Notice how you feel that stress somatically (within your body). Where is it situated in your body? Rate that stressful feeling from zero to ten (zero being not stressful and ten being extremely stressful).

3. Set an intention to reduce those stressful feelings.

4. Using the four fingers of your right hand, start tapping on the 'karate chop' point.

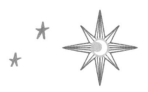

5. As you tap, repeat to yourself three times: 'I feel stressed and accept how I feel'.

6. Focus on how you feel about the stressful event. Continue tapping five times on your meridian points: the crown of your head, the inner point of each eyebrow, the sides of both eyes and under the eyes, the philtrum beneath the nose, the chin, collarbone and under each arm.

7. As you tap, repeat to yourself, 'My stress'.

8. Take three deep breaths when you finish. On a scale of 0 to 10, how do you feel now? End by expanding your emotional freedom with a positive statement: 'I manage stress with ease and confidence'.

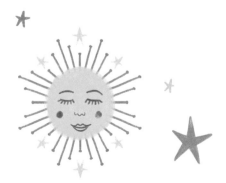

The stress I feel most is

The way I feel after EFT

How I use EFT in my everyday life

A Wild Workout

Scientists have discovered that when we work out in a greenspace (for instance, a park, garden or forest), our brain releases endorphins, reducing stress and improving our mental health. Several studies have found that the mental health benefits we get from being active outside last longer than when we work out in the gym.

Find an outdoor workout that you enjoy such as walking, cycling, running, skating, or anything that appeals to you as long as you are moving your body. If you live in a town or city, go for a walk along a tree-lined street, find a community garden to stretch in or a city park for runs.

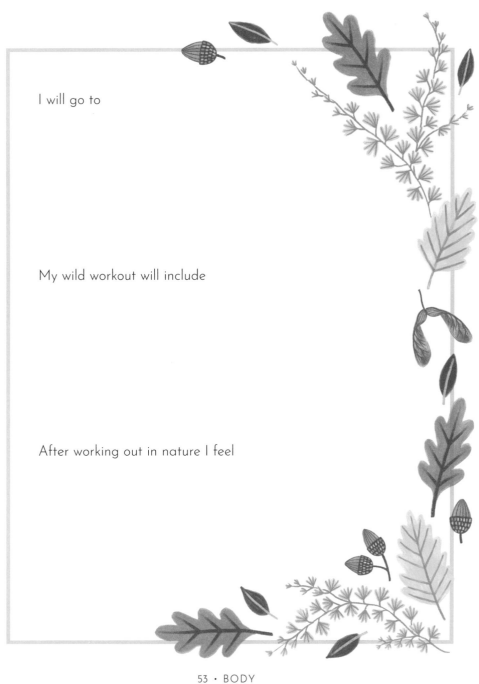

I will go to

My wild workout will include

After working out in nature I feel

Recharge with Superfoods

Hectic schedules mean that we often forget that recharging our energy is just as important as getting stuff done. This is 'sacrifice syndrome', a term coined by Case Western Reserve professor, Richard Boyatzis. Those external pressures lead us to skip meals, forget to refuel or grab the nearest thing to hand when we are hungry.

A rich source of antioxidants, minerals and vitamins, superfoods are an easy way to restore your energy. Easily accessible (and portable) examples of superfoods are red berries, quinoa, oats, green tea, cacao, leafy greens such as kale, spinach and romaine lettuce, chia seeds, nuts and flaxseeds. Incorporating superfoods into your diet will help you to refuel effectively.

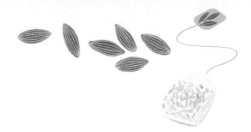

Superfoods to energize me

Superfoods I can prepare in advance

Superfoods I can eat on the move

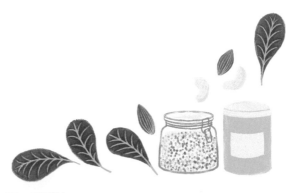

Sleep Soundly with Dinacharya

In Ayurveda, *dinacharya* is the act of creating a daily self-care regime and means 'activities of the day' in Sanskrit. Where better to begin than sleep, the bedrock of a healthy life. Sleep hygiene was developed in the 1970s as a means of tackling insomnia. Today it's used to help people develop good sleeping habits. Decades of research has shown that a sleep hygiene routine that includes the following steps will help to optimize sleep.

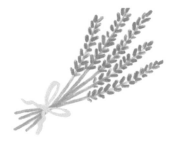

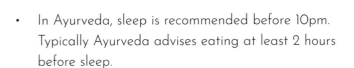

- In Ayurveda, sleep is recommended before 10pm. Typically Ayurveda advises eating at least 2 hours before sleep.

- Create a wind-down routine an hour before you go to bed: turn off devices, sip a bedtime herbal tea and relax. Be consistent with the time that you go to bed each night and the time you wake up.

- Make sure your sleeping area is uncluttered and ensure your bedroom is dark and quiet.

- Find a way to let go of the day's stress. If something is pulling at your attention, write it down on a piece of paper and leave it there. You could also try relaxing with an essential oil. Ayurvedic practices encourage inhaling gentle aromas like lavender or vanilla to ease you into a good night's sleep.

Before bedtime I can relax by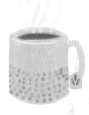

I can improve my sleep hygiene routine by

I commit to waking at the same time every morning at

My sleep routine

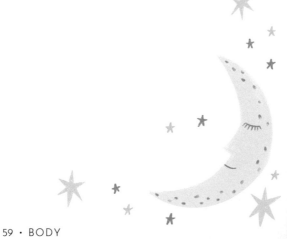

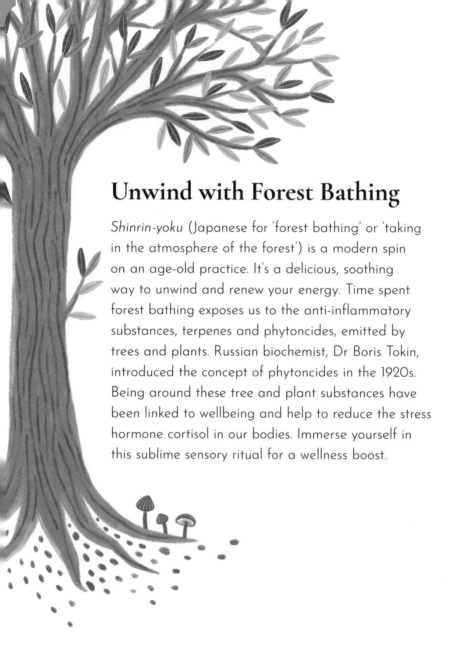

Unwind with Forest Bathing

Shinrin-yoku (Japanese for 'forest bathing' or 'taking in the atmosphere of the forest') is a modern spin on an age-old practice. It's a delicious, soothing way to unwind and renew your energy. Time spent forest bathing exposes us to the anti-inflammatory substances, terpenes and phytoncides, emitted by trees and plants. Russian biochemist, Dr Boris Tokin, introduced the concept of phytoncides in the 1920s. Being around these tree and plant substances have been linked to wellbeing and help to reduce the stress hormone cortisol in our bodies. Immerse yourself in this sublime sensory ritual for a wellness boost.

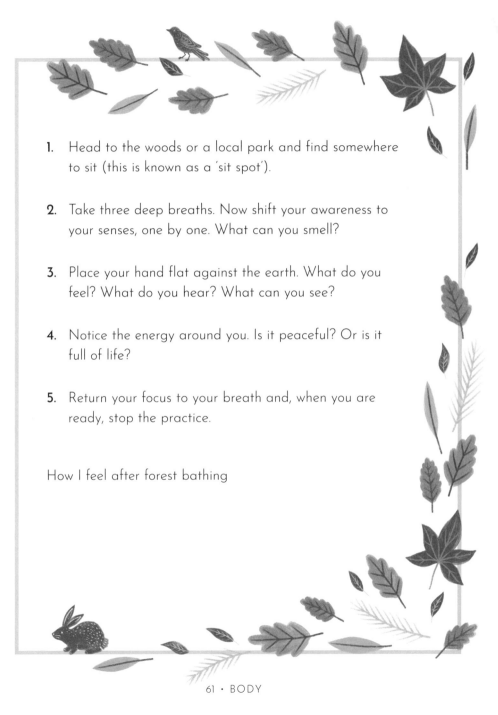

1. Head to the woods or a local park and find somewhere to sit (this is known as a 'sit spot').

2. Take three deep breaths. Now shift your awareness to your senses, one by one. What can you smell?

3. Place your hand flat against the earth. What do you feel? What do you hear? What can you see?

4. Notice the energy around you. Is it peaceful? Or is it full of life?

5. Return your focus to your breath and, when you are ready, stop the practice.

How I feel after forest bathing

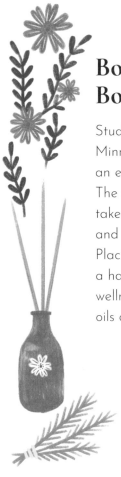

Boost Your Mood with Botanical Diffusion

Studies at the School of Nursing, University of Minnesota have found that botanical aromas have an enormously curative effect on our wellbeing. The natural aroma of plant-based compounds can take you from feeling frazzled and frayed to calm and soothed, thereby supporting your wellbeing. Placing essential oils in a diffuser or a few drops on a handkerchief can have a powerful place in your wellness practice. Why not explore different essential oils depending on your mood and needs?

- Rosemary to help you focus

- Citrus to lift your mood

- Lavender and vetiver to soothe your mind and body

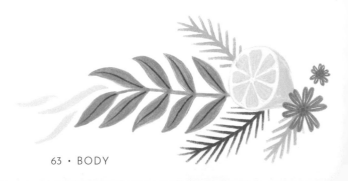

I am energized when I use

I feel rested when I use

I am uplifted when I use

Shower Meditation

Your early morning shower is the perfect time for meditation. Bringing awareness to daily routines is a great way to practise mindfulness. A shower meditation doesn't demand that you dedicate any additional time. Just step into the shower and you are good to go. This self-care ritual is also a wonderful opportunity to channel a positive mindset into your day.

1. Before you begin your shower, take three deep breaths.

2. Feel the warmth of the water on your skin. Notice the sensations of each droplet against your skin.

3. Listen. What do you hear?

4. Bring your focus to the scent of your shower gel or soap. What aromas are here, right now?

5. Is it possible to imagine any tense or stressful thoughts that arise being rinsed away?

6. Dry off and set a positive intention for your day.

My positive intention is

Mindful Morning Sun Ritual

Saluting the sun as it rises each day is an ancient ritual. In Sanskrit it is *Surya Namaskar*, the name for the sequence of yoga poses involved in a sun salutation. For centuries, cultures around the world have created physical practices to greet the new day and celebrate the life-giving sun. You don't need to be a yoga expert to connect with the rhythm of nature at daybreak.

Create your own morning ritual, connecting with the earth to balance and centre yourself. Whether it's facing the sun to feel the warming rays, stretching and meditating, or incorporating existing ancient practices like a sun salute, your ritual will be unique to you.

I feel ready to begin the day when

I will greet the day by

My morning ritual is

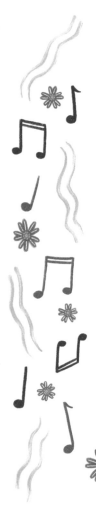

Soft Living

Soft living is an emerging wellness trend. It encapsulates slowing down and taking time to simply be. 'Soft lifers' recognize the importance of enjoying life mindfully and more consciously. Prioritizing wellness and mental health, this way of life supports balance in all things.

Living softly aims to minimize stress. Moreover, it's sustainable, focusing firmly on meaning and purpose rather than possessions. Rejecting the daily grind, advocates of soft living focus on what they enjoy. Eschewing productivity hacks and the pressure to rush from one task to another, they opt for a simpler life. This is living on your own terms.

My values are

How I can align my values with my everyday life

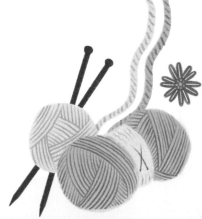

Ways I can find time to do the things I love

Mindful Eating

Eating is often something that we do while we're engaged in another activity. It could be while we are working, watching TV or scrolling through social media. Researchers at the University of Birmingham discovered that we consume more calories when we're distracted. What's more, because our attention is elsewhere, we barely taste our food. They have discovered that mindful eating helps us to make healthier food choices, reduces impulsive eating and lowers stress.

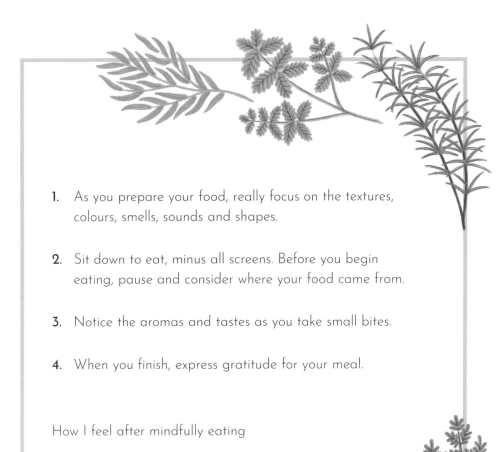

1. As you prepare your food, really focus on the textures, colours, smells, sounds and shapes.

2. Sit down to eat, minus all screens. Before you begin eating, pause and consider where your food came from.

3. Notice the aromas and tastes as you take small bites.

4. When you finish, express gratitude for your meal.

How I feel after mindfully eating

Fika

The Swedish concept of *fika* (pronounced 'fee-kuh') embodies relaxation, restoration and self-care. A noun and a verb, it translates into 'coffee break'. Think of *fika* as a wellness ritual. A pause in your day when you come back into balance with your favourite drink, a nourishing snack along with company that nurtures your soul.

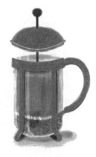

Fika isn't done sitting at a desk chugging through your workload. Think of *fika* as focused calm rather than multitasking with a drink. Researchers at the University of Oregon found that multitaskers were less able to focus, all the more reason to down tools for this Nordic break. Relax and reconnect once, twice or several times during your day with *fika*.

1. Set an intention to have *fika* (and schedule in a time to do so). There's no need to rush.

2. Choose a favourite cup or mug and drink which energizes or calms you, along with an enjoyable and nourishing snack.

3. Find a place for your *fika*, which makes you feel restored and relaxed. It could be a local café, a park, or somewhere peaceful at home.

4. If you feel like company, find time to take *fika* with someone who helps you to feel relaxed.

Afterwards I feel

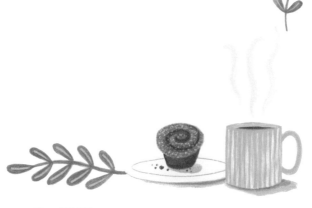

A Perfect Morning Routine

While it's tempting to snooze through the alarm, mornings present the perfect time to establish a self-care routine. Research by Dr Katherine Arlinghaus at the University of Minnesota found that creating a routine helps us to manage stress and anxiety. That's an easy win if you have a stressful day ahead of you.

A routine of self-care welcomes your mind, body and soul into the new day. Whether you think of it as a ritual or the perfect morning routine, by setting an intention for your day, stretching, meditating or sitting with a mug of herbal tea, it will set you on the right track for the rest of your day.

My perfect morning routine is

As I wake up, I feel grateful for

My intention for the day is

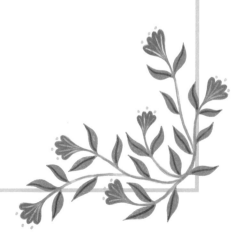

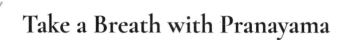

Take a Breath with Pranayama

Practised for over 5,000 years, *pranayama* are powerful Ayurvedic exercises used to control the breath and restore balance. Bringing mind and body together in unison, they possess a plethora of wellness benefits, including better sleep, reduced stress, increased mindfulness, relaxation and focus.

Consciously connecting with your breath is an empowering way to come back into the present moment. Breathwork is potent. It regulates the nervous system and your emotional state. The stillness it provides aids resilience, self-awareness and transformation. When you need to remain anchored, this practice is the perfect vehicle to bring you back to your innate power.

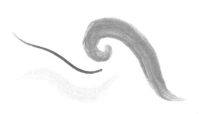

Nadi shodhana pranayama exercise

In Sanskrit, *nadi* means energy channel and *shodhana* describes the act of purification. Also known as alternate nostril breathing, this ancient practice will calm your mind and quieten anxious thoughts in times of stress.

1.   Ask yourself: 'How do I feel?' Find a comfortable, upright position with your feet flat on the floor.

2.   Inhale and exhale naturally, once, without changing your natural breathing rhythm.

3.   Exhale and place your right thumb on your right nostril, closing it.

4.   Inhale slowly through your left nostril for a count of four.

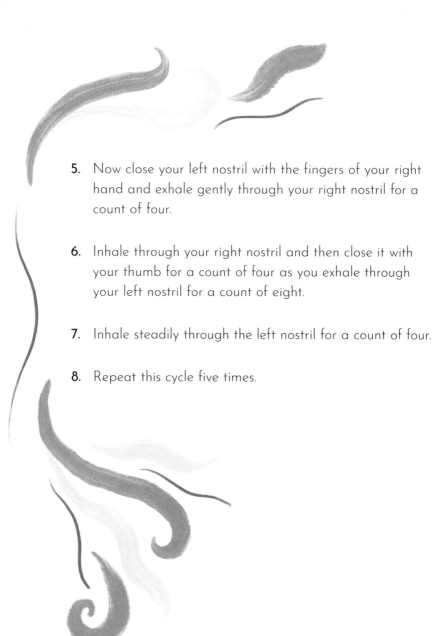

5. Now close your left nostril with the fingers of your right hand and exhale gently through your right nostril for a count of four.

6. Inhale through your right nostril and then close it with your thumb for a count of four as you exhale through your left nostril for a count of eight.

7. Inhale steadily through the left nostril for a count of four.

8. Repeat this cycle five times.

Afterwards I feel

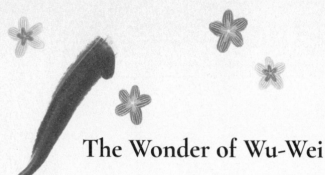

The Wonder of Wu-Wei

In the ancient philosophical text the *Tao Te Ching*, Chinese philosopher Lao-Tzu wrote of *wu-wei*, loosely translated as 'inaction' or 'doing nothing'. *Wu-wei* is something of a paradox. Sometimes by approaching life with a non-striving state of mind, we can accomplish more, authentically connecting with our innate truth and power.

So where could you channel a *wu-wei* mindset and become effortless? This state can only be achieved by being still and slowing down. When we live in harmony, no longer trying to control and force life to bend to our will, a natural rhythm emerges. Only then are we in flow, aligning with magical, universal energy.

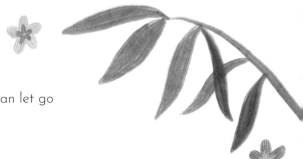

Areas in my life where I can let go

The ways I can step away from busyness and create more flow

Actions I can take to create a more *wu-wei* approach to my day

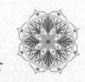

Self-heal Using the Principles of Reiki

An ancient Japanese form of spiritual medicine, reiki purports to use the transfer of universal energy or life force for the purpose of healing. Reiki consists of two Japanese words, *rei*, meaning universal life and *ki*, which means energy. It's the free flow of energy that is used to promote wellness. While reiki is usually performed by a reiki practitioner, you can use these principles for your own self-care.

Dr Mikao Usui is credited with creating reiki in Kyoto during the 1920s. His 'Usui system' is still used around the world today. Researchers at the University of São Paulo suggest that reiki reduces stress, anxiety and pain.

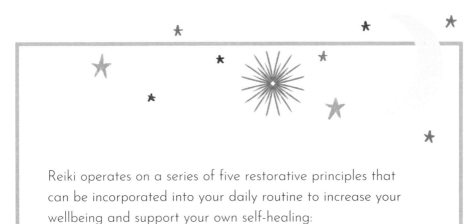

Reiki operates on a series of five restorative principles that can be incorporated into your daily routine to increase your wellbeing and support your own self-healing:

- Just for today, I will not be angry.

- Just for today, I will not worry.

- Just for today, I will be grateful.

- Just for today, I will do my work honestly (be true to myself).

- Just for today, I will be kind to every living being.

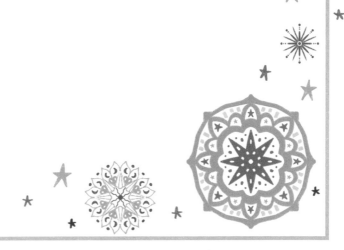

1. I will make time to release anger by

2. Strategies that I can use to minimize worry are

3. My daily gratitude practice consists of

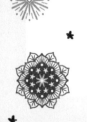

4. I set the intention to be true to myself by

5. I commit to being gentler with myself and others by

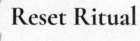

Reset Ritual

Rituals are powerful symbolic practices that are carried out on a regular basis. Many rituals have roots in ancient wisdom traditions and countless human experiences incorporate rituals as markers of life, collectively and individually. Considered sacred actions for centuries, they also serve as a symbolic reminder of what's important to us. Researchers at Harvard University have demonstrated that creating and taking part in rituals can lessen anxiety, increase our efficacy by reducing performance anxiety and uncertainty as well as increasing happiness.

A grounding reset ritual is the foundation of greater wellness. It will help restore calm throughout the day and is the perfect way to familiarize yourself with the power of rituals.

1. Set a time for your reset ritual.

2. Create a space where you won't be disturbed.

3. Ask yourself: 'What do I need, right now, in this moment to reset my wellness?' Trust your intuition. It might be a deep breath, feeling your feet connecting with the ground or an energizing herbal tea.

Notice what you feel physically, emotionally and mentally as you reset.

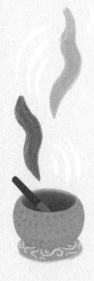

A Healing Sound Bath

Sound is a powerful tool that has been used for thousands of years in many cultures to connect human consciousness with universal energy. Today, sound baths are used as an alternative therapy, working on the body's energetic field to induce deep relaxation and reduce stress. Himalayan singing bowls have been used around the world as a potent form of sound healing for centuries.

A spiritual sound bath with singing bowls is believed to help you connect with different levels of consciousness. You'll need a pre-recorded Himalayan sound bath (there are many available on YouTube), headphones, a comfortable space where you won't be interrupted, a blanket and a pillow to rest your head on.

1. Lie down on the floor. Get into a comfortable position, with your pillow supporting your head and a blanket for warmth. Begin the sound-bathing track.

2. Settle into a gentle breathing rhythm: in through your nose and out through your mouth.

3. Allow the sound waves to wash over you. Experience the energy of the sound as it refreshes, recharges, renews and rejuvenates you.

4. If you feel an energetic block in your body, focus your breath in that area, inviting the sound to clear it. With each exhalation release any stagnant energy.

5. Settle into a natural breathing pattern again. You don't need to do anything, simply be in the moment.

6. When your sound bath is over, slowly roll onto one side before getting up. Have a glass of water handy so that you can hydrate your body.

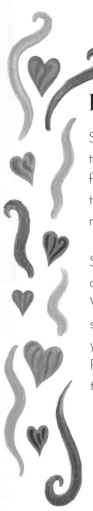

Practise Self-love

Self-love is more than skin deep. It involves being true to yourself and your needs. This incorporates everything from recognizing how unique you are and committing to your own wellness, to eschewing self-sacrifice in the name of keeping others happy.

Self-love is a powerful energetic force. When we love ourselves, we change the frequency of our energy. We begin to attract people, work and situations that support that love. Practise self-love by speaking to yourself as though you are talking to a dear friend. Replace self-criticism with a different dialogue, saying to yourself, 'I accept myself as I am' and 'I am enough'.

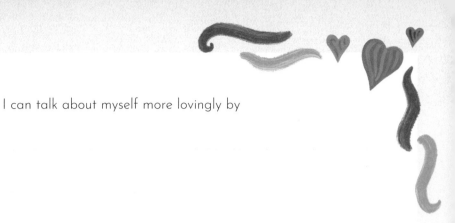

I can talk about myself more lovingly by

How I can prioritize myself and my happiness

Ways I can show myself love

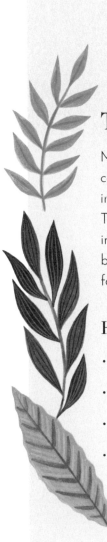

The Healing Power of Mantras

Mantras help us to access our inner strength. They connect to our inner compass, the part of us that intuitively knows how to respond to any challenge. Think of a mantra as a prompt to tap into your internal power. Recite your chosen mantra at the beginning of the day or call upon specific incantations for support in difficult situations.

How to use a mantra

- Ask yourself what you need.

- Set an intention.

- Place your palms over your heart area.

- Recite your mantra.

Something I want to invite more of into my world is

My morning mantra

My mantra in times of stress

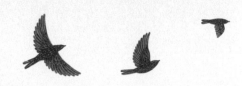

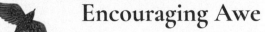

Encouraging Awe

Professor Dacher Keltner, founding director of the Greater Good Science Center, discovered that a daily dose of awe is good for you. Contemplating something that takes our breath away makes us happier, healthier humans. One study by Keltner even found that people who experienced wonder and awe had lower levels of interleukin 6, a protein that helps your body regulate immune responses.

We have a sense of awe when we recognize the sacredness of life. It's a feeling of reverence, inspiration and wonder. You can get a sense of awe in everyday life by watching a sunrise or sunset, listening to music, reading a great book, or simply being in the presence of an act of kindness.

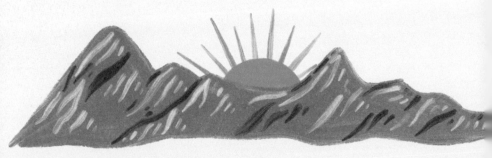

Natural landscapes where I experience wonder

Music and films which inspire awe

Art and literature that fire my imagination

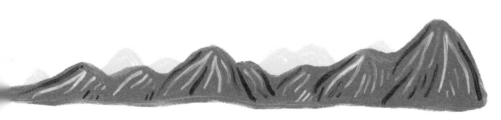

Stop and Stargaze

The external instability and environmental upheaval that is taking place in the world around us is often reflected in our inner world. This is one of the reasons that eco-anxiety is on the rise.

Connecting with nature is soul work. Ancient wisdom traditions recognized that we are inextricably linked to the natural world. We're part of it but we've lost that connection over the centuries, leaving us unable to sense our true place in the universe.

Studies at Harvard School of Public Health show that reconnecting with nature protects our mental health and helps us to connect with our natural environment – an important first step in beginning to protect it. We can start to reconnect with the universe and our place in it by taking some time to stargaze.

1. Wait for a clear night and step outside or open a window. Set an intention to connect with the vastness of the universe. Take three deep breaths and notice the air that you're breathing in.

2. Tune into your senses. Do you detect an aroma or taste in the air? Wood smoke, the scent of grass or something else? What do you hear?

3. Lift your gaze to the sky. What can you see?

4. Are there any emotions present right now? Whatever you feel, allow yourself to experience it without judgement.

5. Allow yourself to be still. See if it's possible to connect with the energy of this vast, beautiful universe. Offer gratitude to the earth and the sky.

Embracing your Shadow Side

Swiss psychiatrist Carl Jung famously noted that 'what we resist not only persists, but will grow in size'. He developed the concept of shadow work, as a way of focusing on the 'shadow self' (the parts of the psyche we keep hidden). When we accept ourselves fully, shadow and all, we can let go of trying to be perfect.

For Jung, the shadow side contained all the parts of ourselves that we shrink away from, suppress or deny. It's everything that we reject and, usually, the very thing that we find annoying and frustrating in others. We can't see it because we're not consciously aware of it. For example, feeling envious of a friend's career success might tell us something about our own aspirations that have yet to be realized. The shadow side of envy can be acknowledged without judgment and used instead as motivation to commit to setting goals for yourself around those aspirations.

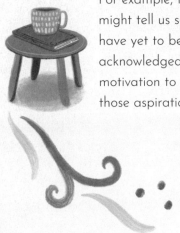

Find a safe space to journal where you won't be disturbed and make yourself comfortable. Pour yourself a cup of calming tea, play music that soothes you, and centre yourself as you bring a non-judgemental attitude to this exercise. Choose an area that you would like to work on.

A part of myself I reject or suppress

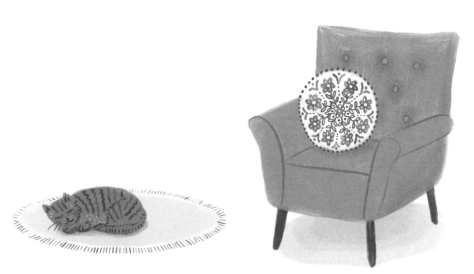

My reflections on what is causing me to feel/act this way and how it impacts my life (Note: if it helps, draw the shadow.)

How I can embrace this shadow part of myself

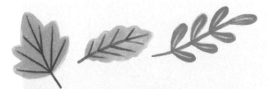

Reconnect with Barefoot Earthing

This supremely calming, stress-reducing practice has been used around the world for centuries. Native American, Indian, Aboriginal Australian and Taoist ancient wisdom traditions all recognize the importance of physically attuning to the ground. Touching the earth with the soles of our feet grounds us and connects us to the natural energy of the universe. Research at the University of California suggest that earthing soothes us, reduces inflammation and improves our mood.

Find a park, lawn, forest, beach or garden. Remove your footwear and stand or walk barefoot. Feel your body connecting with the earth.

Sensations I notice

Before barefoot earthing I felt

Afterwards I feel

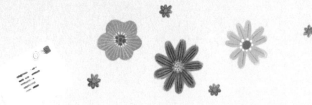
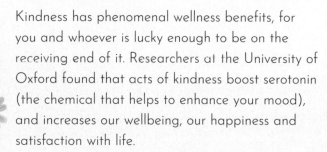
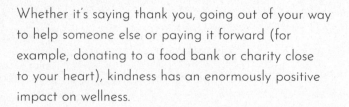

Pay it Forward with Kindness

Kindness has phenomenal wellness benefits, for you and whoever is lucky enough to be on the receiving end of it. Researchers at the University of Oxford found that acts of kindness boost serotonin (the chemical that helps to enhance your mood), and increases our wellbeing, our happiness and satisfaction with life.

Whether it's saying thank you, going out of your way to help someone else or paying it forward (for example, donating to a food bank or charity close to your heart), kindness has an enormously positive impact on wellness.

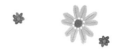

I will begin by offering kindness to myself by

I can show gratitude to

Small acts of kindness that I can practise every day

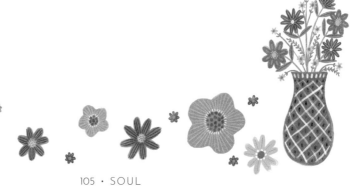

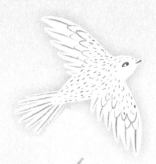

Nature Meditation

When your spirit is low and you're feeling stressed and depleted, meditating on nature will bring you back into balance. Researchers at Colorado State University discovered that when we're listening to sounds in nature, we experience a significant reduction in cortisol, the stress hormone that sends our bodies into a tailspin. Our blood pressure lowers and we're better able to focus. We also feel more connected to each other, the planet and the universe.

To mindfully rewild yourself, step out into nature, open a window or listen to the sounds of nature on YouTube.

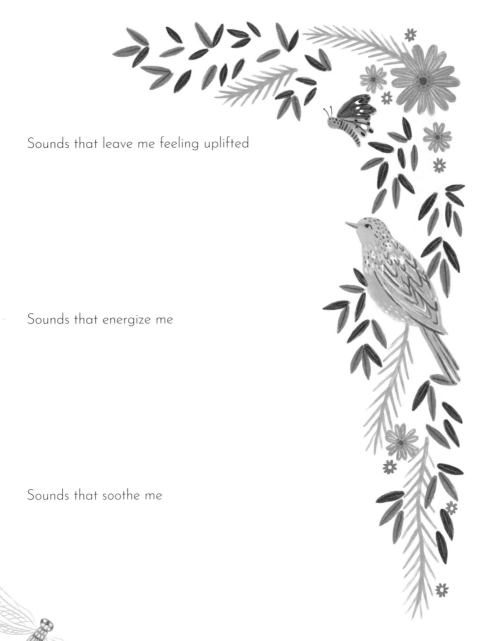

Sounds that leave me feeling uplifted

Sounds that energize me

Sounds that soothe me

Discover Dreamwork

Dreamwork is a spiritual practice based on the work of psychiatrist Carl Jung. He believed that dreams are the unconscious making itself visible. In dreamwork we explore the symbols, images and narratives that appear in our dreams. Think of dreamwork as a morning meditation, a ritual connecting to another realm, one that informs your daily life.

After you wake, begin to delve into your dream. What happened? Try to remember each detail. Begin to journal, capturing your dream, noticing any images, symbols, people or stories and if they hold any meaning for you. Think about any patterns or themes that are emerging and if there is a connection to your everyday life.

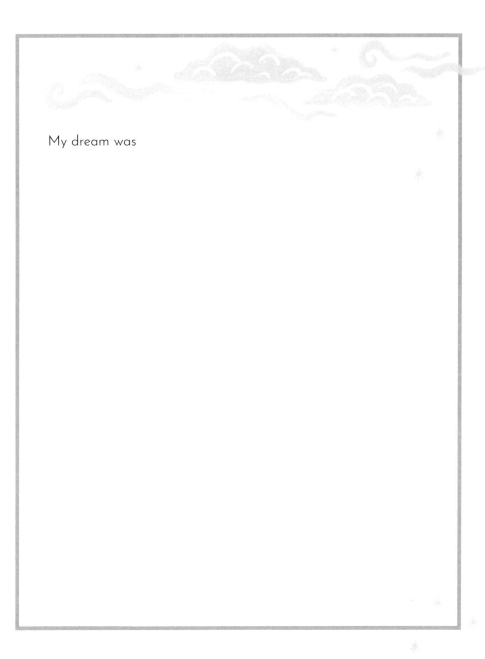

My dream was

Emotions present in my dream were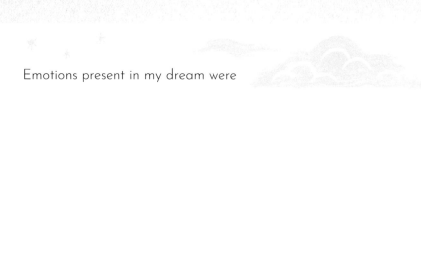

Symbols, themes or patterns that appeared were

The meaning or message that I take from this in relation
to my everyday life

Celebrate Solstices

Around the world, the longest and shortest days of the year have been celebrated across cultures for centuries. Considered a potent time to manifest, celebrating the two solstices honours all that has gone before, paving the way for new goals and dreams. A ritual for marking the turning of the year, the solstice presents a time to turn inward and reflect.

To mark the solstice, find somewhere where you won't be disturbed. Light a candle, and bring a journal to reflect on endings. What has happened over the past six months? Honour everything that has gone before. What are you grateful for? Now shift your focus to new beginnings. What do you wish for?

Choices I will make

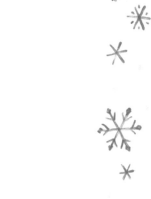

Action I will take

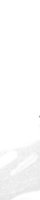

Ikigai

In Japan, finding your purpose or following your joy is encapsulated by the concept of *ikigai* (ee-key-guy). Purpose and meaning are vital for resilience, balance and happiness. *Ikigai* is composed of four elements: what the world needs; what you are good at; what you love; and what you could be paid for. When these four components are combined, the point where they intersect equals *ikigai*, your reason for being. By exploring your inner world, you can begin to connect with your purpose and discover your *ikigai*.

What does the world need?

I'm passionate about and love doing

I can give back by

What could I be paid for?

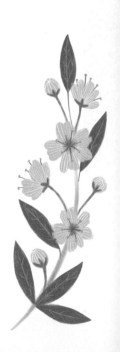

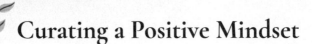

Curating a Positive Mindset

Curating a positive mindset is an incredibly rich spiritual and wellness tool. It helps you to cultivate an energy that is in alignment with the law of attraction. With it you can completely shift your energetic footprint, aligning with the energy of the universe. When you do that, you begin to co-create the life you want, becoming more aware of who you are and the energy that you choose to send out into the world. Deliberately curating the information that you consume is the first step towards auditing your mindset. Reflect on how you feel in each area listed opposite.

How does the media I consume impact me?

Who do I surround myself with?

I will invite positive energy into my life by

Building a Growth Mindset

A 'growth mindset' is a powerful psychological tool, established by Stanford University Professor Carol Dweck, that can transform your mind and soul. A growth mindset helps us to move away from fear and towards a more curious, open approach to life. Instead of playing small and avoiding challenges, developing your mindset expands inner awareness, enabling you to grow and fulfil your potential. Adopting this approach helps us to learn from mistakes, manage failures constructively and do things differently next time.

When you experience challenging life events, nurture a growth mindset by asking: What is the lesson here? What unique opportunity does this present for my personal development and spiritual growth? What can I take away and use? What will I do differently next time?

The ways I can embrace a spiritually conscious life, by making conscious everyday choices that align with my spiritual growth

Dare to be Vulnerable

Conventional wisdom frequently views vulnerability as weakness, but the opposite is true. It takes courage. Vulnerability allows us to be open; to stand rooted in our humanity, directing love towards ourselves even though we know we are imperfect. It's the ultimate form of self-acceptance.

Dr Brené Brown's research found that when we allow ourselves to be vulnerable, we are helping ourselves become more self-aware.

Make a conscious decision to open up to the world instead of hiding yourself. Be compassionate towards yourself and acknowledge that vulnerability takes courage. Release your concern about what others might think and engage in situations that move you out of your comfort zone.

I can show my vulnerability by

I will let go of any expectations of perfection by

I can move outside of my comfort zone by

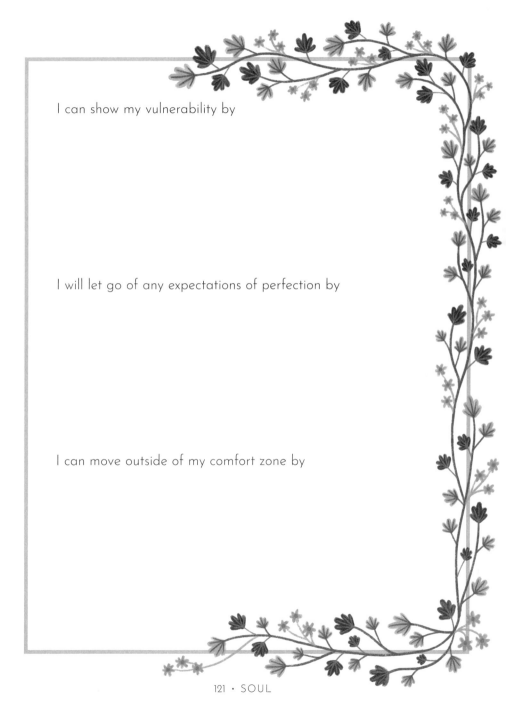

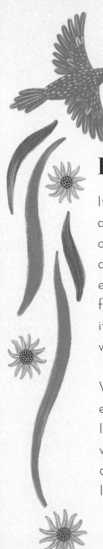

Embrace Letting Go

It's impossible to move through life without hardship and disappointment. No one lives a sterile life devoid of struggle. The Buddhist practice of detachment is a powerful spiritual meditation. Holding onto past events can leave us feeling stuck and unable to move forward. Letting go can feel tricky because sometimes it's tough to move on when things don't work out the way we wanted.

When we let go, we let be. Moving past negative events, loss and disappointment is an act of self-love. It helps us to transform pain and loss into growth and wisdom. Remember, you have the power to let go, to define who you want to be. Detachment is a journey. It doesn't happen overnight.

1. Find a place where you won't be disturbed.

2. Make yourself comfortable and focus on your breath and soften your body.

3. Visualize the situation that you would like to let go of.

4. Now imagine that the sun is burning brightly in front of you.

5. Place the situation into the burning sun and let it go.

6. In each cell of your body, feel the situation disintegrating as it is transmuted by the sun, and let go.

7. Reclaim your sense of balance and feel the power of release.

Is there a way of reframing the event to create a more empowering version that will allow you to grow?

What did this experience teach you and how are you stronger because of it?

Practise forgiveness. We do this for ourselves, to move on and let go, not for the other person. I forgive

The Mind–Body–Soul Connection

At the beginning of this journal, you accepted the invitation to pursue wellness. By now you've realized that wellness is an ecosystem of mind, body and soul. You've been working from the inside out. Focusing on all three components creates a ripple effect in our lives. These traditional remedies, ancient rituals and evidence-based practices can reconnect us to ourselves, each other, and the natural world.

You have discovered potent tools and coping skills for psychological challenges; practices to change your thinking and strategies to shatter limiting beliefs about what you can achieve. You will no longer be at war with yourself. Instead, you will start to develop the ability to feel more positive in every fibre of your being.

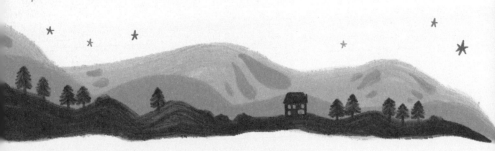

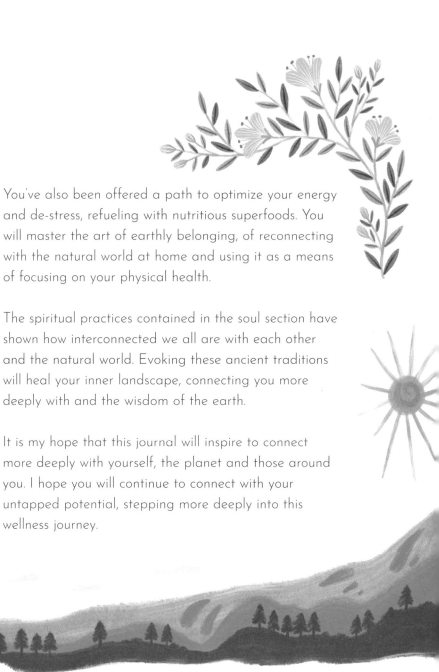

You've also been offered a path to optimize your energy and de-stress, refueling with nutritious superfoods. You will master the art of earthly belonging, of reconnecting with the natural world at home and using it as a means of focusing on your physical health.

The spiritual practices contained in the soul section have shown how interconnected we all are with each other and the natural world. Evoking these ancient traditions will heal your inner landscape, connecting you more deeply with and the wisdom of the earth.

It is my hope that this journal will inspire to connect more deeply with yourself, the planet and those around you. I hope you will continue to connect with your untapped potential, stepping more deeply into this wellness journey.

About Gill Thackray

Gill Thackray is a performance psychologist, lecturer, author and coach, helping organizations and individuals globally, to create conscious transformation and positive change. She has lived and worked with indigenous communities around the world, in Southeast Asia and China. She is a PhD researcher studying eco-psychology and ancient wisdom traditions. She can be found at www.gillthackray.com.

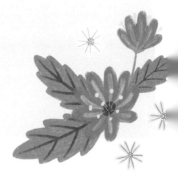